YOUR KNOWLEDGE HAS VALUE

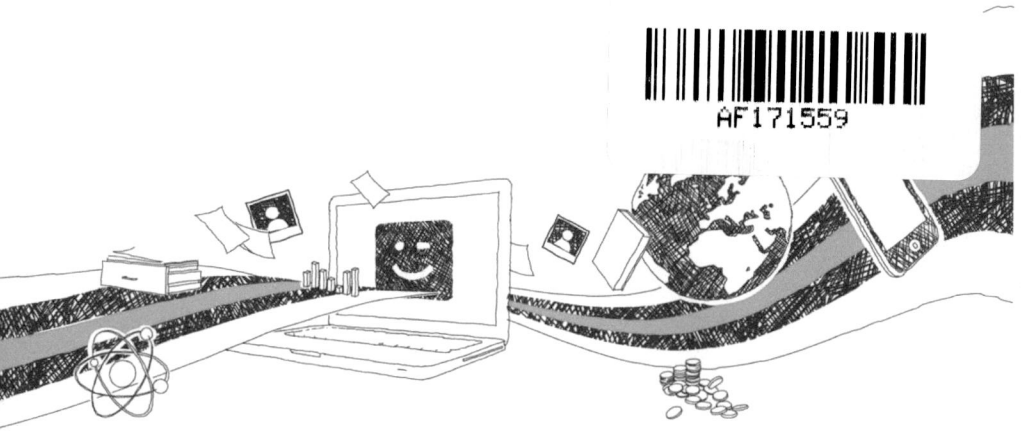

- We will publish your bachelor's and master's thesis, essays and papers

- Your own eBook and book - sold worldwide in all relevant shops

- Earn money with each sale

Upload your text at www.GRIN.com
and publish for free

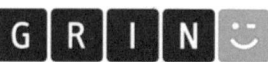

Bibliographic information published by the German National Library:

The German National Library lists this publication in the National Bibliography; detailed bibliographic data are available on the Internet at http://dnb.dnb.de .

This book is copyright material and must not be copied, reproduced, transferred, distributed, leased, licensed or publicly performed or used in any way except as specifically permitted in writing by the publishers, as allowed under the terms and conditions under which it was purchased or as strictly permitted by applicable copyright law. Any unauthorized distribution or use of this text may be a direct infringement of the author s and publisher s rights and those responsible may be liable in law accordingly.

Imprint:

Copyright © 2017 GRIN Verlag, Open Publishing GmbH
Print and binding: Books on Demand GmbH, Norderstedt Germany
ISBN: 9783668595378

This book at GRIN:

https://www.grin.com/document/384454

Patrick Kimuyu

Integration of Nursing Intellectual Capital Theory and Social Exchange Theory in Reducing Medical Errors in Hospitals

GRIN Publishing

GRIN - Your knowledge has value

Since its foundation in 1998, GRIN has specialized in publishing academic texts by students, college teachers and other academics as e-book and printed book. The website www.grin.com is an ideal platform for presenting term papers, final papers, scientific essays, dissertations and specialist books.

Visit us on the internet:

http://www.grin.com/

http://www.facebook.com/grincom

http://www.twitter.com/grin_com

Integration of Nursing Intellectual Capital Theory and Social Exchange Theory in Reducing Medical Errors in Hospitals

Name: Patrick Kimuyu

Inhaltsverzeichnis

Introduction 3

Summary of the Problem and the Potential Middle-Range Theory 3

Middle-Range Theory: Nursing Intellectual Capital Theory 4

Borrowed Theory: Social Exchange Theory 5

Origins of Social Exchange Theory 6

Previous Applications of Social Exchange Theory 6

Applying Social Exchange Theory in Reducing Medical Errors 7

Integration of Nursing Intellectual Capital Theory and Social Exchange Theory in Reducing Medical Errors 8

References 9

Introduction

In retrospect, nursing practice seems to have experienced a remarkable evolution from the classical nursing to evidence based practice. This evolution has expanded the scope of nursing and improved the quality of care to patients. Of great importance is the provision of safe and quality care whose ultimate results are high patient outcomes. As envisaged in core nursing theories and bioethical principles, healthcare is meant to reduce the burden of disease and improve the quality of life of patients. This been the focus in nursing practice, education and research, and the outcome is a transformed nursing practice. Based on this objective, new interventions and nursing guidelines have been developed to promote the delivery of safe and high quality care. Despite this remarkable advancement in nursing care, a number of medical issues have remained as significant barriers in healthcare. Of concern is the problem of medical error which has become a compromise to safe and quality care across the continuum of healthcare system. In principle, medical error is defined from the medical perspective as actions which are done by healthcare providers that can lead to the occurrence of adverse events (Grober & Bohnen, 2005). In other words, medical error is simply a preventable outcome adverse resulting from inappropriate action by a healthcare provider (Van Den Bos et al., 2011). As such, it is apparent that the issue of medical error has an immense implication to nursing practice. Therefore, this report seeks to provide a focused analysis of a mid-range theory and a borrowed theory which when integrated can provide an appropriate solution to medical errors.

Summary of the Problem and the Potential Middle-Range Theory

Across the continuum of healthcare, medical errors have emerged as a challenging medical issue in public care. They occur so often within the clinical setting where healthcare providers encounter difficulties in dealing with the issue. For instance, nurses are adversely affected by the issue of medical errors because it arises as a negative outcome associated with their actions. The fact that nursing practice is based on the core tenets of bioethics implies that any negative outcome associated with their practice is undesirable. Therefore, the occurrence of medical errors in the clinical setting, especially clinical placement, laboratory simulation and nursing practice undermines advancement of the nursing profession. A focused systemic review reveals that the problem of medical errors impairs the quality of care, as well as compromising patient's safety (Grober & Bohnen, 2005). It has both economic and health implications. As the focus of the 21st century healthcare leans towards reducing the cost of healthcare and reducing deaths, medical errors continue to cause deaths which could be prevented. In the United States, it is reported that medical errors cause over 250,000 deaths, annually (Makary & Michael, 2016). Earlier in 2008, preventable medical errors were estimated to cause 200,000 deaths compared to 98,000 deaths reported by the Institute of Medicine in 1998. On the other hand, the cost of medical errors is quite high. Currently, it is estimated that medical errors account for over $20 billion, annually (Andel, Davidow, Hollander & Moreno, 2012). Elsewhere in the UK, medical errors are estimated to cost £2 billion each year (Ker et al., 2010). This implies that the issue of medical errors has an immense impact on healthcare, and specifically on nursing practice due to its association to clinical handovers, nurses' burnout, nursing leadership, and professional competence.

Middle-Range Theory: Nursing Intellectual Capital Theory

In this context, the nursing intellectual capital theory, a middle-range theory has the potential for solving the problem of medical errors within the clinical setting, especially in nursing practice. This theory is designed to address issues related to nursing intellectual capital. In principle, the nursing intellectual capital theory combines nursing human capital and nursing structural capital as the core theoretical concepts. From a theoretical perspective, the concepts exhibit interdependence in nature, and they are perceived to influence both patient and organizational outcomes. As conceptualized by Covell (2008), nurse staffing and employer support for nurse professional advancement promotes nursing human capital which when combined with nursing structural capital produces desirable patient outcomes, as well as organizational outcomes.

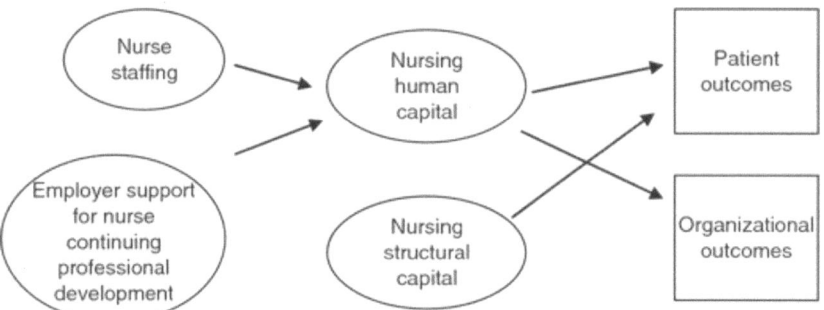

Figure: Components of the nursing intellectual capital theory (Covell, 2008)

Borrowed Theory: Social Exchange Theory

From a theoretical perspective, the issue of medical errors has a significant relationship with nursing knowledge and the social aspect of nurses. This implies that exchange of social resources within the clinical setting can address the problem of medical errors; primarily in nursing practice where nurses' interactions and collaboration with other healthcare providers underpins delivery of evidence based nursing care. Therefore, it is apparent that the social exchange theory is appropriate for solving medical errors.

In principle, social exchange theory presents a sociological approach to negotiated exchanges involved in social change and stability. This theory shares a close relationship to structuralism and rational choice theory. The basic concepts of the social exchange theory revolve around cost and rewards. According to Lambe, Wittmann and Spekman (2001), exchange, as conceptualized in the social exchange theory, is a social behavior that exhibits social and economic outcomes. As such, it is presumed that social exchange generates satisfaction in situations where costs are covered by fair returns. In this case, relationship decisions are based on costs and rewards. As explained by the social exchange theory, costs can be defined as elements of rational life with undesirable consequences to an individual, whereas rewards are the positive returns from a relationship. Overall, this theory has several assumptions related to human nature and relationship. One of these assumptions is that humans are rational beings. The second assumption is that humans avoid punishments and seek rewards. Third, it is assumed that humans use diverse standards in evaluating rewards and costs. Finally, it is postulated that rational life occurs as a process and that relationships are interdependent (West & Turner, 2007).

Additionally, there are several theoretical prepositions that structure human behaviors in the context of rewards and costs. The first preposition holds that behaviors that generate appreciable outcomes tend to be repeated. Second, it is stated that rewarding an individual's behavior promotes its execution. Third, it is postulated that the value of reward diminishes upon subsequent repetition (Cook & Rice, 2013). Concisely, the social exchange theory holds that individuals minimize costs by pursuing rewards.

Origins of Social Exchange Theory

In brief, the social exchange theory was developed by George Homans in 1958. It was then advanced further by Richard M. Emerson and Peter M. Blau who aligned it with the exchange approach within the context of sociology. Consequently, psychologists such as Harold Kelley and Thibaut John integrated psychological concepts into the social exchange theory based on their studies. Similarly, Levi-Strauss had a significant contribution in the development of this theoretical perspective from the context of anthropology where he explained systems of generalized exchange including gift exchange and kinship systems Cook & Rice, 2013).

Previous Applications of Social Exchange Theory

From a critical perspective, social exchange theory has previously been extensively applied in sociology, business and psychology disciplines. However, it is application in interpersonal relationships has gained an unprecedented popularity. In anthropology, this theory helps in explaining cultural ideas and norms (Cropanzano & Mitchell, 2005). Similarly in the business field, the social exchange theory explains diverse aspects in business practices. It extends to work settings where it explains levels of engagement in an organization by employees. For instance, it explains the reciprocal interdependence amongst employees within an organization (Saks, 2006).

Applying Social Exchange Theory in Reducing Medical Errors

In retrospect, it is apparent that the social exchange theory can be applied in nursing to address the issue of medical errors. The fact that it explains self-interest and reciprocal interdependence implies that nurses can improve their practice through the aspect of interdependence. In the one side, it can enhance nurse-nurse interactions, as well as, collaboration with the other healthcare professionals. This can create an avenue for sharing nursing knowledge which, in turn increases nurses competence, one of the key factors associated with medical errors. Second, this theory promotes collective responsibility amongst nurses aimed at achieving positive outcomes, in this case, job satisfaction and high patient outcomes. This way, clinical handover issues which results into medical errors can be minimized within the care setting. In the other side, the adoption of this theory can change the way organizations view nursing knowledge. In the contemporary nursing, knowledge is considered as an essential element for professional competence. As such, healthcare organizations invest extensively in individual development of nurses. However, social exchange theory introduces an advanced perspective to nursing knowledge which is viewed as an exchange resource.

Overall, the adoption of the social exchange theory into nursing practice has a significant impact to a nurse. First, it requires nurses to view others as important parties in professional practice. It can enhance collaboration through interdependence, in order to gain rewards. Second, this theory can change the way organizations reward nurses. It can introduce changes into the reward system leading to improved satisfaction amongst nurses, hence reducing medical errors.

Integration of Nursing Intellectual Capital Theory and Social Exchange Theory in Reducing Medical Errors

From a theoretical perspective, the social exchange theory can be integrated with the nursing intellectual capital theory to solve the problem of medical errors within the care setting. One of the approach through which these theories can be integrated to solve medical errors is adopting nursing intellectual capital theory in addressing issues related to nursing human capital and nursing structural capital, whereas the social exchange theory addresses issues related to nurses relationships including nurse-nurse relationship, nurse-patient relationship and nurse-physician relationship. This integration model can ensure that organizations provide support to nurses and address staffing issues. Additionally, the integrated model can enhance interdependence and satisfaction amongst nurses leading to improved patient outcomes through minimizing costs, including medical errors.

The second approach through which these theories can be integrated to solve the problem of medical errors within the care setting is through the development of a theoretical framework based on the key concepts explained in both theories. Such a framework should consider organizational support to nurses advanced training, staffing and knowledge exchange as some of the main aspects of nursing practice. This framework can address nurses staffing issues, burnouts due to work overload, handovers and professional competence; thus solving the problem of medical errors.

Overall, an integration of these theories into nursing practice can transforms the way organizations view nurses, as well as, reducing healthcare costs as it is hypothesized in evidence based nursing practice.

References

Andel, C., Davidow, S., Hollander, M., & Moreno, D. (2012). The economics of health care quality and medical errors. *J Health Care Finance, 39*(1), 39-50.

Cook, K. S., & Rice, E. (2013). Social exchange theory. In J. DeLamater & A. Ward (Eds.), *The handbook of social psychology* (pp. 53–76). Berlin, Germany: Springer.

Covell, C. (2008). The middle-range theory of nursing intellectual capital. *Journal of Advanced Nursing, 63*(1), 94-103.

Cropanzano, R., & Mitchell, M. (2005). Social exchange theory: an interdisciplinary review. *Journal of Management, 31*(6), 874-900.

Grober, E. D., & Bohnen, J. (2005). Defining medical error. *Can J Surg., 48*(1), 39–44.

Ker, K., Edwards, P., Felix, L., Blackhall, K., & Roberts, I. (2010). Caffeine for the prevention of injuries and errors in shift workers. *The Cochrane Database of Systematic Reviews*, 5, CD008508.

Lambe, C. J., Wittmann, C. M., & Spekman, R. E. (2001). Social exchange theory and research on business-to-business relational exchange. *Journal of Business-to-Business Marketing, 8* (3), 1–36.

Makary, D., & Michael, D. (2016). Medical error—the third leading cause of death in the US. *BMJ, 353*, i2139.

Saks, A.M. (2006). Antecedents and consequences of employee engagement. *Journal of Managerial Psychology, 21*(7), 600–19.

Van Den Bos, J., Rustagi, K., Gray, T., Halford, M., Ziemkiewicz, E., & Shreve, J. (2011). The $17.1 billion problem: the annual cost of measurable medical errors. *Health Affairs, 30*(4), 596-603.

West, R., & Turner, L. (2007). *Introducing communication theory.* New York, NY: McGraw Hill.

YOUR KNOWLEDGE HAS VALUE

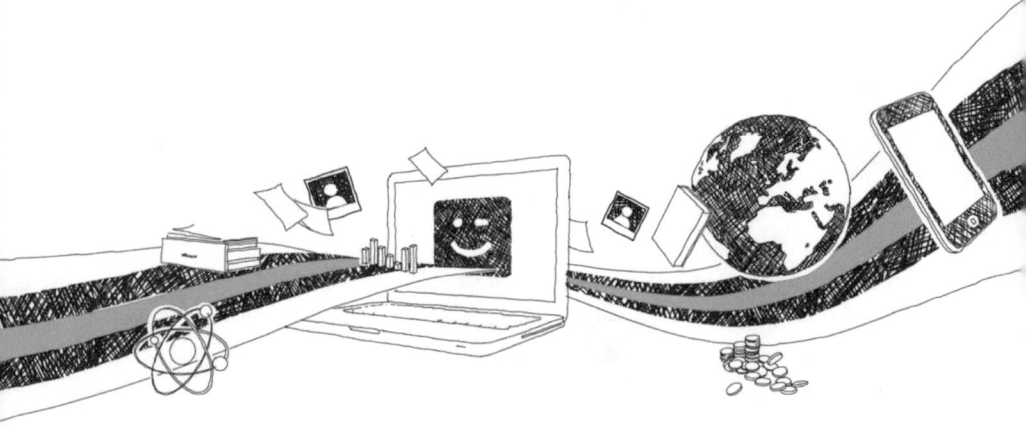

- We will publish your bachelor's and master's thesis, essays and papers

- Your own eBook and book - sold worldwide in all relevant shops

- Earn money with each sale

Upload your text at www.GRIN.com
and publish for free

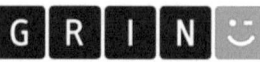